Downward Spiral

A Chat with My Fellow Americans

Sadly Ritten

Fulton Books
Meadville, PA

Published by Fulton Books 2024

ISBN 979-8-88982-210-3 (paperback)
ISBN 979-8-89427-402-7 (hardcover)
ISBN 979-8-88982-211-0 (digital)

Printed in the United States of America

Credits: Many thanks to my wife Andrea, typist Kira, and artist Shelly.

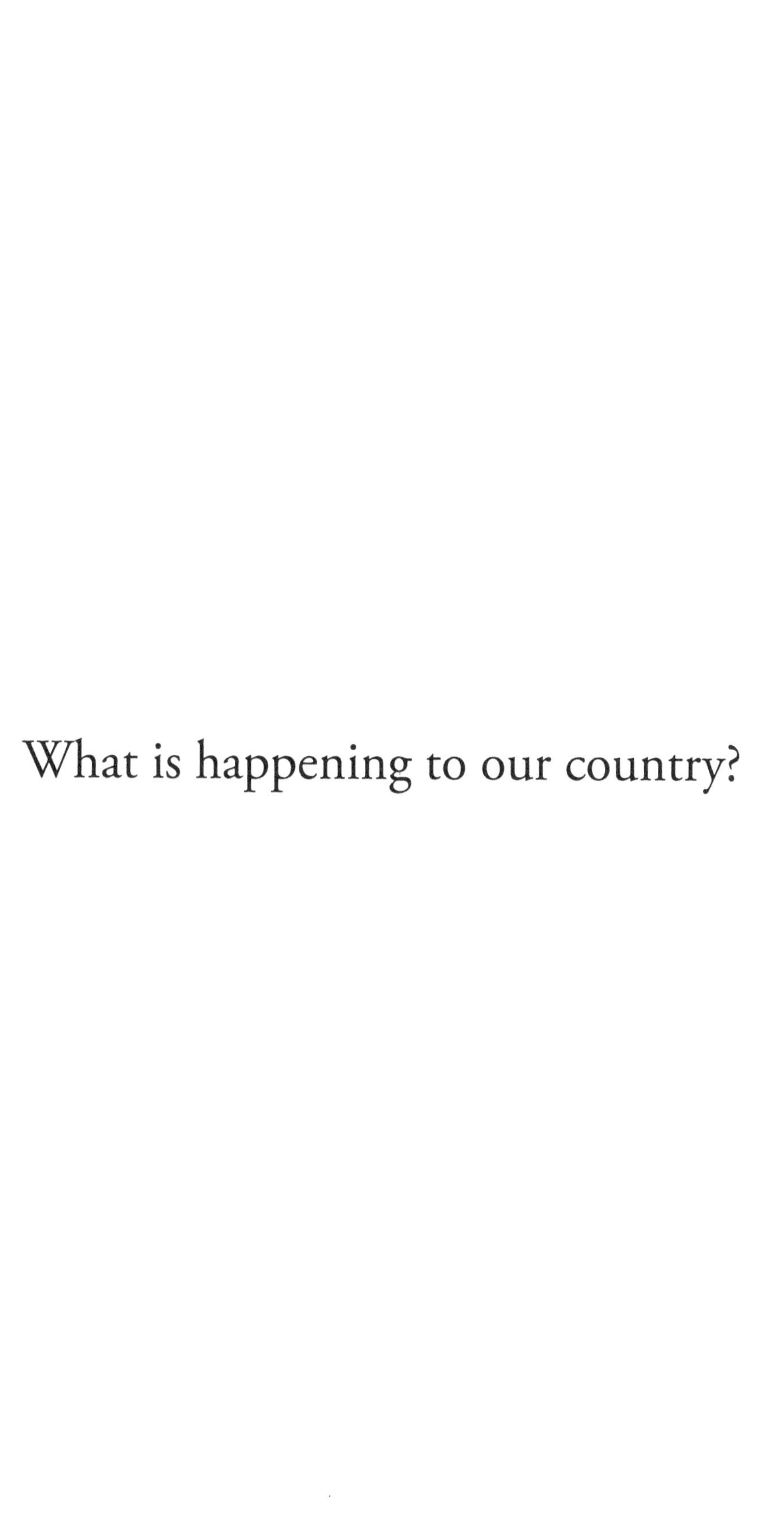

What is happening to our country?

Why read this chat?

1. Our country is portrayed as it actually is.
2. We need to realize facts, whether they be good or bad.
3. We must lead our lives and those of our children and grandchildren in the best way we can.
4. Perhaps we can come up with some solutions to our problems.

Contents

Preface

Sadly, this fireside chat will bear witness to the moral decline of our country. Most of us are aware of what is occurring, but choose to ignore it. Perhaps this is reasonable because there is no stopping the descent, only ups and downs along the way. For the few who have lived long enough to have witnessed the change, this is especially heartbreaking. Please join me in this discussion and form your own thoughts and opinions.

I am not a writer nor a scholar nor a researcher, and certainly not a genius. Neither am I a politician nor a philosopher. I am just an American citizen who served my country in the armed forces and who tried to help my fellow citizens and contribute to the good.

As you read, recognize and remember that *most/all statements are generalizations*; for example, the statement that all white-tailed deer are mostly brown with white tails is false—there are albino deer that are totally white. Many feel that attorneys are primarily interested in making money for themselves, but there are some who honestly serve their clients. And although most doctors treat their patients with excellent care, there are a few who actually cause suffering and harm and some who are obsessed with monetary gain.

Introduction

America, our country, is in decline. We all realize it, but don't want to acknowledge it or speak about it. After all, we have been the number one country in the world for several centuries.

I am just a concerned citizen, especially for the future of our children and grandchildren.

I invite you to join me in a sort of fireside chat. You will certainly not agree with all my thoughts and recommendations, but if you are truly introspective and honest, I think you will agree with many.

Some do not believe in the cyclical theory of civilization, but the decline of many great cultures, such as the Roman Empire, bears witness to the truth. Our country is on its way down the slippery slope, and unfortunately, although there will be ups and down in the coming years, the decline will continue with no way of stopping it. The reason?

The Way It Was

The nature of our society is changing.

When our country was truly great, people were polite and courteous, with friendly greetings and conversations. There was concern for others and mutual respect. Contracts were often agreed upon and finalized with a handshake. There was a lack of vulgarity, and there was a willingness to help others. Family units were the norm, and extramarital affairs and single-parent families were uncommon. Believe it or not, a boy and girl could actually enjoy a romantic date without sex. Most people adhered to our laws, and older citizens were respected. Religious activities were common, and there was respect for our flag and the military members who kept us safe.

There were no smartphones, air conditioners, credit cards, frozen foods, electronics, TVs, or fast-food outlets.

Markers of Moral Decay

Many proclaim that the USA is the greatest nation on earth. However, you may want to obtain and read an interesting *Newsweek* article of August 2010 that proclaimed Finland as "the best country in the world." Our USA rated poorly in many categories, and I doubt we have improved.

Surprised?

Yes, our nation has been great, but look at some of the events we are responsible for:

1. We came to this continent and made it our own. We killed thousands of Native American Indians, took their lands, caused great suffering and death, stole their livelihood, and sequestered them on small particles of land. We stole their freedom. I recall visiting Old Oraibi of the Hopi tribe years ago, where I met and talked with Lily Hamana. She was living in a sparsely furnished hut with a dirt floor. There was little furniture and one cooking pot. As she related how her people were now forced to live on a small reservation, I will never forget the sadness on her face, the depression, the resignation. I was ashamed.
2. We kidnapped human beings from their home in Africa, transported them like animals, and forced

them to serve as slaves. Some were treated inhumanely, and we considered them to be inferior. Many still feel that way. We lost more than 650,000 lives in a civil war trying to rectify this injustice with little success. We tortured and lynched Black people. Become familiar with the Tulsa massacre, recently brought to light.

3. We burned human beings at the stake as "witches."
4. We corralled American citizens of Japanese descent in camps at the beginning of WWII.

Our country's heritage embodies certain ideas. First of all, freedom was at the forefront. We were established as a God-fearing Christian nation, but with religious freedom preserved for all. We were "democratic," meaning ruled by the majority. Of course, this was never true because a candidate for the office of president could receive a majority of popular votes, but lose because of the electoral college—a "representative democracy." A law such as the ACA can become reality through devious means and one vote, despite a large majority of our citizens opposing it.

The United States has the most multivehicle accidents (MVA) involving alcohol, the most drug-related deaths, the highest infant mortality, and the highest number of cases of AIDS.

When did the decline of our great county begin? I think it began right after WWII, the last large moral war. That period was one of jubilation. People were excited, and in my opinion, two factors emerged that were at least partially responsible. Many will not agree with me, and some will be downright angry.

The first was the importation of the Beetles! Their raucous songs, such as "A Hard Day's Night" and "Ticket to Ride," excited the country and youth. The second was Elvis Presley, "the King," with such nonsense as "All Shook Up" and "Hound Dog." Oh yes, were you aware that the King was one of the biggest prescription drug addicts ever? Hail to the King!

These influences began the death of civility and aroused aboriginal feelings. But guess what else happened: the mothers went as batty as the kids!

How do I know this? I experienced it.

Admittedly, after doing their dirty work, both groups produced some decent, mediocre music. I doubt any of the Beatles would have been chosen on the Voice, but Elvis probably would have.

These two groups exemplify one way to become famous, make money, and influence people and cultures. What are your favorite examples of such actions?

Cheap ways to become rich and famous:

Would it be exposing your pubic hair in a movie?

Would it be exposing a breast on national TV during a football event?

Would it be twerking on stage during a formal affair on national TV?

Maybe a comic using foul language initially, then toning it down after the spotlight?

The people responsible for these acts do not deserve our respect or praise, and certainly not our admiration.

Society/Race

Why are we having such problems with the acceptance of African Americans into our society?

Perceived negatives toward blacks:

1. Exaggerated emotional response
2. Different hairstyles and clothes
3. Many obese with big butts and thighs
4. Muddy complexion
5. Assumed low IQ
6. Unique sayings and greetings
7. Visions of people as slaves
8. Body odor different from other ethnicities
9. Opinion of not contributing to society in a positive manner
10. Fear of aggression

But there are other factors that are often ignored:

Psychological:

Things that are white:	Things that are black:
• Daytime	• Nighttime
• Angels	• Grim Reaper
• Wedding dresses	• Mourning clothes
• Clean things	• Dirty things
• Good-weather clouds	• Storm clouds
• Drinking water	• Sewer water
• Salt	• Pepper

Breaker of family:

The father's absence has led to adolescent violence, suicide, drug overdose, obesity, and video games, with lingering effects.

Our environment is getting hotter—fast! We are tempted with all sorts of wonderful things but no plan to pay for them. Many people would rather receive government handouts than go to work.

Sexual attacks and perversions are commonplace and increasing. There is a lack of adherence to our laws—"I'll do whatever I want."

We revere Dr. King and other civil rights activists, we tear down Civil War monuments, and we outlaw the term "nigger." But only one factor will lead to improvement—*time*.

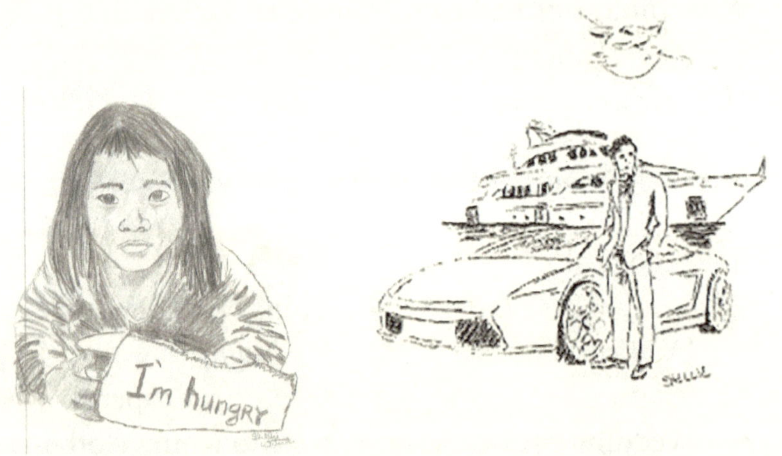

There are two egotistical billionaires spending billions
of dollars to soar into space while millions of children in
our country need food and medical care. Perhaps they
should receive the Humanitarian of the Year Award!

Federal Government

Are we headed for socialism or a dictatorship?

It's obvious that states are losing control to make their own decisions and chart their own course.

It's also very apparent that we are losing our individual rights, including the right of free speech.

The premise of democracy is the rule of the people, by the people. But do we have a democracy? No. We have a representative democracy, which means that someone else votes for us. This system exudes opportunities for political fandangling, for example, districting.

Do you realize that a president can be selected even if a majority of our people are in favor of another candidate? It's not really difficult; add up the votes, and the person with the highest number wins! Admittedly, there is some justification for our present system—a type of fairness.

The electoral college, used since our country was established, seems to favor smaller states over larger ones, but a national popular vote would seem to favor the larger states. You are encouraged to study the college and make your own impressions. It is unlikely to change.

If we chose a popular vote, why not the same reasoning for other decisions?

Obviously, every situation could not receive a popular vote; the Congress could take care of the less important ones.

But perhaps twice a year, the really important issues could be decided by a majority of the people. Some such issues could include gun rights, gay marriages, immigration policies, national debt ceilings, and term limits.

It's obvious the two-party system isn't working. The Congress has a horribly low approval rating, and the two sides are constantly fighting—not even able to come together on small matters, like two bratty fighting children.

A nation divided against itself cannot
stand. (Abraham Lincoln)

Damn the Democrats. Damn the Republicans. Unfortunately, the majority of our elected leaders are a bunch of incompetent goons. Listen to them. (My apologies to the minority.)

Admittedly, the one whom we expected to reconcile the differences was/is either unable or unwilling to do so.

Why not elect our officials by popular vote? It works locally—why not federally? Candidates would first express their credentials and ideas locally, then statewide, and finally nationwide. At each level, candidates would be chosen by popular vote. Also, at each level they would be able to express themselves on public media. The people would soon eliminate the candidates who do nothing but throw feces on their opponents. And think of the billions of dollars that could be saved by eliminating political contributions and raucous rallies—money that could be better utilized, for example, toward repairing our crumbling infrastructure, feeding our hungry children, and providing suitable housing for all.

A fairy tale

There was once a nation on planet Earth that was considered the very best. It had the most wealth, the latest inventions, a low crime rate, mostly nice people who were to rule themselves according to the majority, a justice system designed to protect the innocent, vast natural beauty and resources, and freedom for all, with the opportunity to better oneself.

In order to guide such a large number of citizens, leaders were elected and laws promulgated to guide the course of the nation. The top person selected was the president. There were a number of presidents over the years—some good, some not so good.

In one recent election, a man with very persuasive speech and the ability to influence others—not unlike Jim Jones and Adolf Hitler—won the presidency over another candidate who had extensive experience and enthusiasm.

Well, he didn't really win. A majority of citizens voted for the other candidate, but the electoral system allowed the presidency to go to the influencer. Rule by the people?

Voting is a democratic privilege, a right, and an obligation. While you may think that your single vote doesn't mean much, our vote added to millions of others could mean significant life changes for our country. Unfortunately, only slightly more than half our citizens vote, whereas in some other countries, the percentage is in the eighties.

What a dilemma is immigration! Because we have failed to follow our laws, we have millions of noncitizen immigrants. What shall we do?

Actually the solution is simple. First, close the border; the southern border, of course, since our neighbors to the north have little reason or incentive to become US citizens. Second, all individuals with a criminal record should be deported. Third, all illegal aliens would be given the opportunity to become citizens by demonstrating the ability to converse in English and pass a basic citizenship test. Obviously, the younger set would be well equipped to attain the goals. Older individuals would be tutored locally and given one year to comply. Failure would equal deportation. Done.

ACA is a mess. No one can fault President Obama and/or Hillary Clinton for attempting to provide quality health care to all our citizens. The problem with the plan was the failure to consult all pertinent parties in order to satisfy the majority. One gets the impression that a bunch of clerks sequestered themselves and came up with 2,700 pages of regulations that no one read.

It didn't take long to discover the true nature of a recent president. Consider the following:

Negatives:

1. No military experience—draft dodger
2. No mainstream political experience
3. Thousands of documented lies
4. Defamed other countries, especially Mexico
5. Defamed religions, especially Muslims
6. Inactivity regarding COVID—"hoax" magically disappeared
7. Self-serving, prideful, wrathful, gluttonous, lustful, greedy
8. Supplicant to autocrats in China, North Korea, Russia, and Turkey
9. Withheld Ukraine money until they would announce an investigation into his political rival

10. Sought reelection help from China
11. Adulterer and womanizer—"grab 'em by their pussy"
12. Expressed support for military, then threatened to take away defense money
13. "Musical chairs"—White House loss of good people
14. Disrespect for American heroes, such as John McCain
15. Continuation of horrible government debt: $725 trillion tax cut!
16. Nepotism
17. Ego—perhaps greater than Ellen DeGeneres or Steve Harvey
18. No concern for most; favors rich friends
    a. Rallies that spread disease
    b. Pardons for felons and political buddies
19. Speech via notes
20. Not a good businessman: six bankruptcies, possible tax and finance violations
21. Low diplomatic capability
22. No role model
23. No promised health care plan
24. Considered by some to be incompetent, vindictive, mentally unstable, misogynistic, homophobic, racist, traitorous, and an egomaniac

Is this the kind of person you would want your children and grandchildren to be?

I did hear a rumor, however, that the queen invited this president for tea and trumpets.

Then a terrible viral pandemic came to the country, causing thousands of deaths and horrible suffering. Despite competent medical advice from various sources, this president declared the disaster a "hoax" and said it would soon go away. He refused to follow medical advice and promoted various "cures" that included a medicine of no value and the taking of substances that were not only worthless, but potentially dangerous.

By not shutting down the whole country initially, many, many people have suffered and died. He continued to "open the country," "it is what it is."

It's wonderful to get all these things for free—but *someone has to pay for them!*

We have no money.
We are over $30 trillion in debt!
And we give money to those who loan money to us!
(and no one apparently gives a damn)

Incidentally, you might like to know where our nation's dollars come from:

1. Foreign governments, chiefly Japan and China
2. US banks and investors
3. The federal reserve
4. State and local governments
5. Mutual funds
6. Insurance companies
7. Savings bonds
8. Tax dollars

Suggested requirement for a president:

1. Age 35–70, US citizen
2. College degree
3. Free of criminal history
4. Military experience (UMT acceptable)
5. Outstanding moral character/humility
6. Good health
7. Honesty
8. Unbridled enthusiasm
9. Respect for our constitution and laws

Some of the factors we need to consider are the following:

1. Terrorist attacks (foreign and domestic)
2. Corrupt politicians
3. Loss of a common language
4. The welfare state violent entertainment
5. Rise of pedophiles and child abuse
6. Unchecked debauchery
7. Class warfare
8. Taxation and the national debt
9. Trade deficits
10. Mass shootings

We know, and the world knows, that we possess the greatest military machine known to man. We also have thousands of war casualties: missing arms and legs, burn scars, mental disabilities, the list goes on and on. And for what? Since WWII, nearly 120,000 Americans have died fighting in places like Korea, Vietnam, Iraq, Afghanistan—none of them with clear-cut victories.

The only justifiable war since WWII was our involvement in Kuwait, and that upon the request of their government. Vietnam was a total disaster and a national disgrace, and look at Iraq, Syria, and Afghanistan.

I couldn't believe that we invaded Iraq, on a presidential whim and against the advice of our allies. But Dickie and Donnie, along with a weak president, prevailed.

At the time of the election, the American people made it clear that they wanted our troops out of Iraq, and the president agreed. Well, we finally pulled out some of our troops after several years, and then the forces were sent to Afghanistan! What did we accomplish? Nothing. These countries have been fighting for centuries and will continue to do so for many more.

You cannot legislate morality.

Sex

For the purpose of our discussion, "sex" will refer to the following:

A male and female meet and find a mutual physical, and perhaps emotional, attraction. They begin with gazing into each other's eyes, then comes "foreplay," which may consist of kissing and touching.

Then a suitable place is sought: this may be a bedroom, an office, a vehicle, or on the kitchen table.

The desire to join bodies becomes more intense, clothes are removed, and various acts of feeling, kissing, and tonguing follow. The male's penis rises to the occasion, and in various positions, the penis is inserted into the female's vagina amid an orgy-like panorama of panting, groaning, and other utterances.

This is followed by the "dry off," when both partners feel extreme fatigue and sigh, and they reflect on the previous events. Some feel a cigarette is appropriate at this time, and they may take a nap. They are both left with a sticky mess.

This instinct was given to us with the primary purpose of propagating the race, and therefore it should be pleasurable. But have we taken undue advantage of this?

You may want to review the biblical teachings regarding the relationships between men and women:

1. Sexual activity was designed to further the race.
2. The concept of becoming "one flesh."
3. Marriage as a lifelong commitment.
4. Adultery is considered a sin.

Many of these concepts may be found in Mark 10, Matthew 19, and Ephesians 5:

1. Sex on impulse or lust is wrong.
2. Sex with love and commitment is right.

You are encouraged to review these teachings. Look around you. Sex is everywhere:

1. Between consenting adults, hopefully with love
2. Outside of marriage
3. With relatives

4. With animals
5. As part of initiation rights and party games
6. As physical and psychological relief
7. As a therapeutic modality
8. By respected bodies, even presidents
9. By the clergy
10. In various positions
11. In public places
12. At mile-high altitudes
13. In various forms, as sadism and masochism
14. In return for money or favors
15. As an attention getter
16. Maybe a power play, as for blackmail
17. With members of the same sex
18. As an instant gratification
19. As a greeting
20. On TV and social media

Well, let's keep going. How about these:

1. A monthly sex day, where everyone can have sex with whomever they want?
2. Sex for admission to shows, clubs, political positions, and other advantages?
3. Sex huts, where people can run in for a quickie. Prices could be kept reasonable through punch cards; one session free for every ten?
4. Distinctive award for the greatest number of conquests or maybe the number of different partners?

Where will it end?
There are also other considerations and consequences.

With no birth control, infants can be born without the knowledge and desire of sexual partners, resulting in unexpected and possible unwanted children—many without a father figure, many without a support system (including financial).

The father's absence can lead the child to obesity, violence, suicide, and substance abuse.

Any male who impregnates a female should bear responsibility for the products of conception. This would include marriage, but would mandate that the male would bear the financial burden of the resultant products of conception. If he is not able to do this, he should be become a state worker with his wages used for the necessary support of the mother.

Another factor is the transmission of venereal diseases such as gonorrhea, syphilis, chlamydia, and HIV, which can occur without protection. Billions of dollars are spent on the treatment and prevention of these illnesses.

The single mom

There should be no single moms, with the exception of partner death, extreme incompatibility, and certain physical conditions.

Percentage of US births to unmarried females:

    1980 – 18 percent
    1990 – 28 percent
    2000 – 33 percent
    2010 – 41 percent
    2019 – 40 percent

Rape is one of mankind's most vicious crimes. Do you consider removal of a penis cruel and unusual punishment?

Consider the following:

There was once a typical small American village with a small population. This is a story of two people.

Mary was a nine-year-old schoolgirl—cute, full of life, smart, nice to everyone. She was very friendly to everyone, loved the local playground, and had joined the local girl scouts. Her parents both worked and struggled to pay the rent and provide food for the table. They were good people and loved their little girl.

Also in the town lived Bruno, a middle-aged brute man who dressed sloppily, had no job, was antisocial, and disliked by most of the townspeople. He had been involved in sexual acts, but had never been arrested or diagnosed with a mental illness. He was known to ogle girls when they passed.

One morning, Mary got dressed, ate breakfast, slung her backpack on her shoulder, and headed for school after saying goodbye to her mother and father. Her path took her on a narrow dirt road with woods on either side. She hummed a little song as she skipped along.

But then Bruno jumped out of the woods in front of her. His face was flushed, his body menacing. Mary was frightened, and she screamed and tried to run, but Bruno caught her and dragged her into the woods. Mary struggled to escape, but he was too powerful. Bruno threw Mary down on the ground and tore her clothes off. When she began to scream, he stuffed her panties into her mouth and slapped her face hard. Tears ran down her face. She struggled and writhed as he forced her legs apart and unzipped his pants. Bruno forced his large member into Mary's tiny body, causing tearing of her flesh and much bleeding.

When Bruno had finished, he realized what he had done, and there was no other course than to strangle her quivering body, which he did, before running away. Mary's body was found two days later.

Is this not cruel and unusual?

Removal of the penis would not only prevent a lecher from repeating his crime, but would serve as a powerful deterrent to others.

Homo/LGBTQ

Homosexuality is a difficult topic.

Many of us have many friends, and many develop very close relationships, which is fine.

Gay people have been discriminated against and harmed both physically and mentally for years, although this has changed considerably over the past few years.

We must also recall that the HIV epidemic was largely spread—if not originated by—homosexuality, resulting in billions of dollars for medical care.

Let's look at the situation from a physical standpoint. The human body was designed so that continuation of the race would be fairly simple and pleasurable, and easy to attain.

The male's penis was designed to fit inside a vagina, not to be shoved into the rectum or the mouth and licked like a lollipop.

Sexual activities were designed to further the race, and although pleasurable in most instances, they were not for self-gratification, stress relief, or a good time.

Let's also examine the Bible's teaching regarding homosexuality:

1. Leviticus 18:22 and 20:13 state that, "You shall not lie with a male as with a woman; it is an abomination."
2. In 1 Corinthians 6:9–10, it states that, "Men who have sex with men and other acts will not inherit the kingdom of God."

Other biblical references can be found in these passages, as well as others:

1. 1 Timothy 1:10
2. Revelation 21:8
3. Romans 1:26–27

There are biblical scholars who believe that the scriptures are misinterpreted, that sexual intercourse between men (or women) is not a sin, and that love transcends all. You are encouraged to further investigate this topic.

Personally, I find homosexual acts disgusting. The sight of two men kissing on the lips makes me want to vomit. But please understand—I grew up in a time when men were men.

Other sexual aberrations will not be discussed, but

1. practitioners should not be objects of discrimination,
2. public money should not be used for purposes such as changing one's sex, and
3. God's judgment is yet to come.

Other situations we must confront include these:

1. Cyber flashing
2. Teen sleepovers
3. Affairs
   a. Mark Sanford
   b. Eliot Spitzer
   c. Anthony Weiner
   d. Arnold Schwarzenegger
   e. John Edwards
   f. David Petraeus
4. Sex videos
5. Prostitution

Crime/Guns

We have many things in abundance in our country; one of them is crime, and another is guns. Let's review some statistics:

- The incarceration rate in our country is approximately 743 per 100,000. The incarceration rate in Canada is approximately 131 per 100,000.
- The annual cost of violence is approximately 12 billion dollars.
- Ten to twenty-four percent of prison inmates are mentally ill.
- Approximately 2.8 million Americans have schizophrenia.
- In 2008, the Supreme Court confirmed gun rights for individuals.

- Americans draw their firearms in self-defense ±200,000 per year.
- There are more than 300 million guns in the USA.
- Forty percent of gun sales are made by unlicensed private dealers.
- The Eddie Eagle GunSafe program of the NRA is a useful way to teach firearm safety to our youth.
- Background checks are supported by 90 percent of Americans and 85 percent of gun owners.
- There were 251 mass shootings leaving 520 dead and 2,000 wounded (January 1–August 5, 2019).
- ATF Operation Fast and Furious—a giveaway program.
- Less than 5 percent of the world's population owns 42 percent of firearms.

Guns are used more to protect life than to take life.

There is anger, contempt, and intolerance for each other—we are meaner, nastier, and more cruel.

How about the influence on our citizens, especially the younger sets, of violence and blood gushing seen in video and electronic games?

Psychologists, and especially the perpetrators of this gore, assure us that there are no adverse effects on our children. But we all know better, don't we?

Have you noticed thousands of our children are killed, injured, or disabled every year because of gunfire. People are nastier and more likely to react in a violent way when upset.

Highways

Do you ever get frustrated while driving?

Do you see drivers far exceeding the speed limit, cutting in and out of traffic lanes, failing to use turn signals, flipping the bird, operating under the influence of drugs (yes, alcohol is a drug), texting and primping while driving, running red lights, passing on solid lines?

In the USA, there were over 3 million automotive injuries and over 3,860 automotive deaths in 2020. The numbers continue to rise.

All these acts reveal a total disregard for the very laws that are designed to protect us. What is worse, many have little respect for the law enforcement officers attempting to keep the highways safe. This situation is a national disgrace. Consider the following solutions:

First, all traffic laws should be reviewed and altered appropriately:

1. Reevaluation of all speed limits.
2. No more 55 mph limit on open roads in good condition. Speed realistic for road conditions. All traffic lights timed the same so that drivers could more accurately assess whether to proceed through the light.
3. No more 35 mph signs for construction that isn't even there.
4. Stop signs of two types:
    a. Slowing and looking both ways before proceeding.
    b. Total stop, no motion.
5. Raising the minimum driving age to eighteen years old.

Second, strict enforcement of all non-speeding violations—for example, running a red light, one of the most dangerous and potentially fatal acts that is unfortunately occurring more and more.

Third, all speeders exceeding 10 mph over the posted limit in any place and any time would be referred to a Reminder Center (RC)—a reminder to obey our laws. Local RCs would be established. The typical building would be sealed tight. After removing their clothes, the lawbreaker would be supplied with a rear opening gown and a hood and would be attached to a pole. The gown would be opened, and an appropriate number of whacks or lashes applied to the buttocks. He or she would also be responsible for any monetary fines and penalties. An audience would be allowed, but no recording devices of any sort. Potential recorders would be severely punished and imprisoned for five years. The only exception from this punishment would be provided by a physician's excusal. All these cases would be reviewed, and if found unjustified, the physician would receive the same penalty, thus eliminating the "my buddy, the doc" scenario.

Within a few months, only regional centers would be needed. Problem solved.

Since this is not likely to happen, a second option is available:

Making the punishments meaningful. No more $50 fines and twenty-point penalties.

Dogs learn by rewards, humans by the threat of punishment:

1. A $50 fine for every mile above the posted speed limit (e.g., $600 for going 82 mph in a 70 mph zone).
2. For more severe offenders, such as running a red light or passing a school bus with flashing red lights or a DUI, a $1,000 fine and placing their vehicle in impound for several months.
3. For very serious acts, in addition to a judge's sentence, seizing the offender's vehicle and selling it at auction. Any remaining balance would be the responsibility of the owner. Then a ban of driver's license for at least a year and hours of community service.

You might think that your chances of getting caught is pretty slim—there are few police officers for the millions of drivers. But wait!

A core of observers would be established. These people might consist of previous law enforcement officers, retired military, etc. They would be equipped with cameras that would register the speed of a vehicle and record the license plate, as well as the time and date of a motor vehicle violation. This information would be valid in traffic court.

There are certain acts that are particularly aggravating:

How about a tractor trailer on a two-lane road passing another one that is travelling 0.1 mph slower, thus tying up traffic for perhaps ten miles?

Or the impatient driver in the lane behind you flicking his lights in your rearview mirror, even though you are travelling at the posted speed?

Drivers using the time waiting for a red light to turn green by texting, applying lipstick, etc.

The "snake maneuver"—veering from lane to lane to gain perhaps several seconds?

We need courtesy and civility in our driving habits.

Motorcycles

Imagine that you just took delivery of a brand new shiny $40,000 motorcycle with all the possible accessories. The salesman beamed as he said it will go over 200 mph, but he says, "drive safely," and off you go, zooming down the highway. 50, 60, 70, 80. Wow! What a thrill! Wonder if it'll go 90.

So down the road you go, roaring happily along, completely oblivious to the stench and roar left behind for others.

And as you go racing down the road, a car who didn't see you, because of your small size and excessive speed, pulls out in front of you in your lane. No time to lay 'er down, you hit the side of the car. *Smash!* You remember flying through the air, about two hundred feet. In just a split second, you see a fleeting image of your wife and two great kids and then *splat!* You are now impaled in a tree with a limb protruding through your abdomen. Your arms and legs are dangling uselessly, your face beyond recognition. There is blood everywhere.

But you don't mind—you're dead. Another suicycle disaster.

It is amazing that anyone will straddle a seat above an engine with two attached wheels without any protection whatsoever.

> Motorcycle statistics:
> 2017: 5,172 died in crashes (14 percent of
>   traffic deaths)
> 2018: 4,985 died in crashes (14 percent of
>   traffic deaths)

You are twenty-nine times more likely to die in a motorcycle crash vs. a passenger car and nine times more likely to be injured.

Ten most common causes of motorcycle accidents:

1. Speeding
2. Driving under the influence
3. Lane splitting
4. Sudden stops
5. Inexperienced drivers
6. Left turns
7. Dangerous road conditions
8. Motorcycle defects

So if you really digest the facts, it's obvious that anyone who cares about self, family, and friends; anyone who agrees that highway safety is important; anyone who is considerate of others; anyone with common sense and with a brain larger than a snail *would have to agree that motorcycles and ATV-type vehicles without adequate passenger protection should be outlawed.*

Should this not occur, the following steps might be taken:

1. Motorcycle riders should have their own insurance exchange, separate from the general auto pool. If they can afford the cycle, they can afford the premium.
2. In case of an accident involving a motorcycle, the "other party" would have to be 100 percent responsible for a successful judgment against them.

How about rules for pickup trucks?

1.
2.
3.
4.
5.
6.

That's right, there are none. They do whatever they damn please.

Health

Look around at our citizens. What do you see?

Fat. Let's review the following realities:

Only a tiny fraction of obese people have a valid reason for their excess fat (e.g., a thyroid problem).

Recently, a male citizen apologized to an overweight TV personality because of her weight, stating that she was a poor example for America's youth. She is, and he should not have backed down.

There is plenty of fat in the United States of America to make tallow for enough candles to light up the whole country for a week (an estimate!).

But let's get serious. What are some of the effects of all this fat?

A fat person takes up the space of two to three people, exceeding the maximum capacities of maternity rooms, elevators, seats, and similar places, and takes more than their fair share of weight restrictions. Airlines may have to reconfigure their seat sizes and weight limits.

Many fat people engage in meticulous grooming, but obesity tends to accumulate debris and odor—especially in the private areas.

More cloth is needed to cover the massive surface areas.

One could sustain injury if unfortunate enough to have a three hundred pounder fall on you. Fat riders put a strain on a horse's back and an auto's tires.

Okay, enough. Let's examine the true effects of obesity:

1. High blood pressure
2. Heart problems
3. Arthritis—degenerative joint disease
4. Cancer—kidney, gallbladder and pancreatic, heart, endometrial, ovarian
5. Liver problems
6. Strokes
7. Sleep apnea
8. Mental illness
9. Infertility
10. Sexual dysfunction

The obesity rate in our country is currently about 36 percent, including 17 percent of teens, and is predicted to rise to 44 percent by 2030. We are the most obese nation in the world.

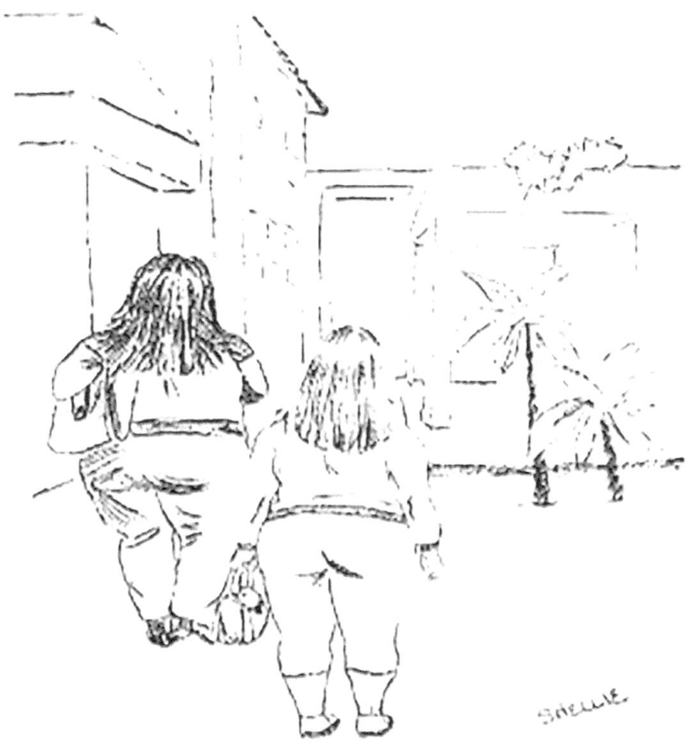

It costs over \$1,400 per year to treat obesity, and over \$700 per year to treat a diabetic. Obesity-related illnesses cost 147 to 210 billion dollars per year.

If an obese person is stigmatized, this may lead to binge eating, depression, low self-esteem, poor body image, anxiety, and suicide.

In our country, 69 percent of the population is overweight, 36 percent are obese, and 32 percent of adolescents are overweight or obese.

Many obese patients with high blood pressure and/or diabetes can improve their health, and sometimes eliminate their problems simply by reducing weight.

Some of the factors that contribute to our rising obesity problem are increased serving sizes, readily available fast-food franchises, constant bombardment of advertisements for calorie-rich foods, a more sedentary lifestyle, emotional states, habit, and social conformity.

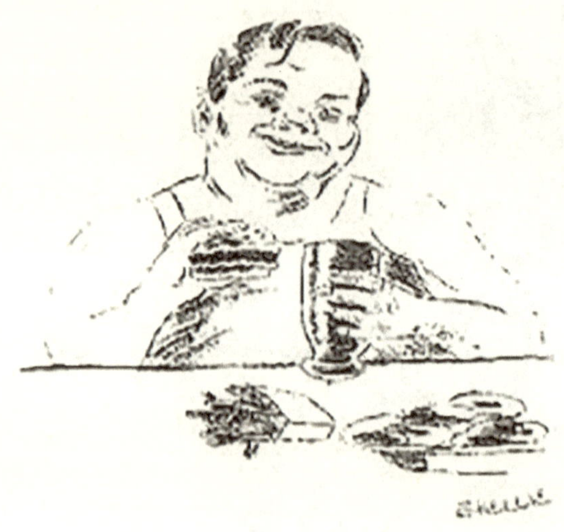

The foods with the most addictive response are sugar, fat, and salt (three main culprits are ice cream, chocolate, and pizza).

There is some justification for being obese, as low thyroid function, genetic factors, and certain mental states. But most of us just don't give a damn.

Some people spend huge sums of money on various plans and diets that promise weight loss. They're "doing something," *but for the majority of us, we simply must recognize the dangers of obesity, and self-discipline to a reasonable daily calorie intake (usually around two thousand) of healthy foods coupled with a moderate exercise program.*

Help and guidance for both of these is readily available from local health sources or online. For example, there are at least two breakfast cereals that can provide nearly all your essential daily vitamins and minerals. No need to spend money at the local nutrition store.

Maybe you feel that these people have a right to live in any manner they choose. And perhaps you're right—certainly if only they are affected. On the other hand, the remaining "normal" population must shoulder a large burden, primarily in increased healthcare costs. Is this fair? Is this a form of stealing?

Reflect for a moment of the hundreds of "entrepreneurs" who have become rich from this group of people.

How many fad diets, dietary supplement, exercise machines, exercise programs, operations?

How many work? How much work over the long haul? How much money wasted? Yeah. Is obesity a disease? I don't buy it.

The tragic fact is that this large group of people lacks the will, the fortitude, and the self-discipline to control their own lifestyles.

It is just so damn simple; eat a well-balanced diet, avoid excess calories, and exercise!

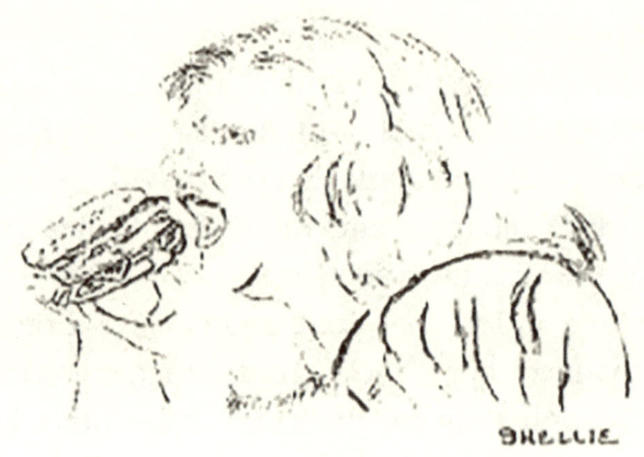

How about all the supplements available in the health food stores? There are vitamins, minerals, probiotics, pills, and liquids for stamina, mental health, well-being, better eyesight, most anything. Perhaps this money would be better spent on healthy foods.

And how about "power drinks"? Add a little caffeine, an attractive bottle, and a good advertising campaign and you have a great rip-off. Many of us support the originators and manufacturers of these gems, but to whose advantage? Well, theirs—we make a few people very rich. The truth is, with a few exceptions, a healthy person eating a healthy diet does not need dietary supplements. But keep on buying them—millionaires are counting on you.

We Americans gorge ourselves repeatedly with tons of high-calorie and fatty foods, often to the point of heartburn and nausea.

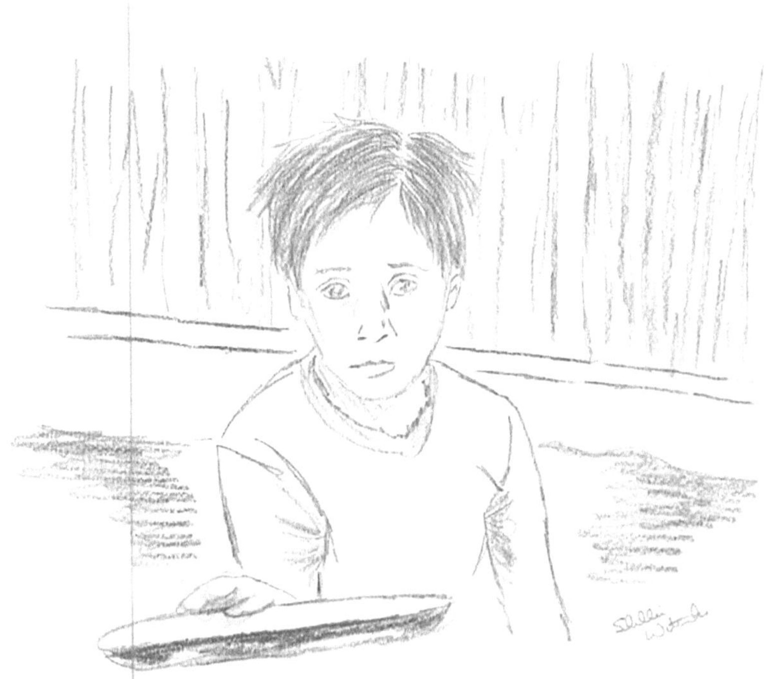

He is saying, "Could you spare a slice of bread?" You say that this lad must be from another country—a poor one at that. No, he is in our country, and there are millions just like him. Maybe that next time we stuff our stomachs to the limit, we will see the image of this poor hungry boy and do something about it.

In addition, people should avoid or at least minimize the intake of biscuits and rolls, breads, sugar, white potatoes, and any fatty foods. Healthier foods include lean meats (e.g., fish, pork, or chicken without skin), low-fat dairy products, raw vegetables, most beans, and fruits.

And eat less!

Oh, yes—have you heard of the new miracle drug? It's called Curall. Surely, you've seen the add on TV. It is guaranteed to cure all your illnesses, from the common cold, to heart attacks, to cancer, even mental problems.

Ask your doctor if Curall is right for you; maybe he or she will prescribe it in place of the many medicines you are already taking.

However, if you experience any of the following side effects, discontinue the drug at once, and call your doctor—even in the middle of the night:

- Drowsiness
- Dizziness
- Headache
- Fatigue
- Muscle cramps
- Excess burping or flatulence
- Loss of hair
- Swelling
- Vision problems
- Palpitations
- Pain (anywhere)
- Nausea and/ or vomiting
- Depression/ suicidal thoughts
- Anxiety
- Rash
- Fainting
- Flushing
- Impatience
- Insomnia
- Tremors
- Excessive sweating
- Loss of appetite
- Decreased sex drive
- Weakness
- Excess salivation
- Tingling sensation
- Tooth discoloration
- Overgrowth of hair
- Ringing in the ears
- Constipation
- Shortness of breath
- Cough

- Diarrhea
- Weight loss and/or gain
- Superboner (lasting more than 4 hours)

- Dry mouth
- Frequent urination
- Urine discoloration
- Skin discoloration itching
- Abnormal dreams
- Easy bruising
- Bleeding

- Fat redistribution
- Gait disturbances
- Hot flashes
- Warm feeling
- Hiccups
- Change in voice/hoarseness

- Fever
- Restlessness

- Skin lesions
- Change in taste sensation
- Menstrual irregularities
- Paranoia
- Aggressiveness
- Seizures

- Wheezing
- Increased thirst
- Prolonged wound healing
- Personality changes
- Nasal congestion
- Hives feeling of doom
- Cold extremities
- Asthenia

Okay, this is ridiculous, but the point is we take too many medications, many of which are totally unnecessary. This leads to drug interactions, adverse effects, allergic reactions, and increases the need for medical care. Unfortunately, many drugs are prescribed because we demand them.

We are bombarded by ads for medication on TV or in published newspapers and magazines, and even on the Internet.

One example is the TV ads for Viagra and Cialis that air frequently. Their advertised benefit is for patients with erectile dysfunction, or ED. We all know it's because men want to attain a superboner.

The drug companies' actions are greedy, unprofessional, dishonest, and (oh yes) profitable.

However, the real tragedy is *we Americans must have our pills!*

Some thoughts:

Health care is not a right—check the Bill of Rights.

Quality health care should be available to everyone.

All citizens should contribute toward their health care.

People who abuse themselves (such as drug addicts/substance abusers, obesity, and smokers) must assume more responsibility for their care

End of life

What should happen to us when our physical capacities are gone and our mental status has plummeted from ten to one? Do you realize that we spend 56 percent of our health care dollars on patients over fifty-five years of age, increasing as age progresses?

The answer is not simple. We like to keep our relatives and friends for as long as we can, but this often causes more suffering for everyone, including the newly departed. Millions, if not billions, are spent on terminal cases.

Obviously, these decisions are difficult and must take into account the desires of the patient as well as the family. Every situation is unique and must take into consideration all physical, mental, and spiritual aspects.

I believe that quality of life is most important.

Smoking

Smoking is one of the worst vices ever. No one should smoke or be exposed to smoke. Smoking has deleterious effects on your body, including the lungs, heart, skin, and the immune system.

Among our other addictions, such as nicotine, alcohol, and sex, we must consider drugs of abuse such as cocaine and fentanyl.

ce of overdoses every year. To consider these actions as a disease is somewhat irrelevant. If we didn't use them, we wouldn't have to fight their importation.

Also, addicts had a choice—*they could have and should have refused the first contact with these substances.*

But in America, we believe in second chances. After an initial failed rehabilitation, the addict deserves another try. But if this fails, the person should be removed to a remote island—the group being provided with basic essentials for life. The only exceptions would be those people whose addiction began with legitimate use of painkillers of surgery; they would receive specialized care.

Military

Yes, our leaders tout our military triumphs. They praise our soldiers, lay wreaths, spotlight a surviving spouse, and blow trumpets. Yet there doesn't seem to be enough money to properly compensate and care for our casualties. There is even talk of decreasing military benefits. Is it not sad and embarrassing that civilian groups have to pass the plate for our military members?

How would you like to live in a 4 × 8 hut in a humid jungle with temperatures hovering above 100±? No shower, no change of clothes, no toothpaste or soap. A handful of rice daily dumped on the floor, a cup of filthy river water twice a day. Surrounded by insects, dangerous animals, and the smelly bodies of your fellow prisoners.

How about being placed in a four-foot bamboo cage and lowered into filthy, stinking jungle water for hours on end? Would you like to be immobilized and have your fingernails ripped off as part of an interrogation?

Would you like to go on patrol and enter a cave with highly poisonous snakes hanging from the ceiling by their tails? One bite on your arm or leg would require cutting off the limb within minutes to avoid death.

Or how about swinging spikes coated with feces, sure to cause a life-threatening infection and a painful agonizing death?

During the entire twenty-four hours, the constant threat of an attack—guns, bombs, rockets. Sleep very difficult and only with total exhaustion. You're walking across a field when suddenly, there is a terrific *boom*. You find yourself lying on the ground; you look down and see you have no legs and the stumps are bleeding. You were a victim of an IED. Maybe you'll survive.

Since the enemy was known to plant bombs on women and children, approaching them under order to kill and firing, whether or not they were loaded, then having to live with yourself for the rest of your life.

If captured, penned up in a tiny cage with little to eat or drink, no toilet facilities, and torture sessions to obtain information. Water dripping, electrical stimulation, sleep deprivation, and other things too gruesome to relate.

Most veterans who experience these tragic inhumanities do not want to discuss them. Our military members did their duty and must live with the sequelae. And we benefit.

The next time you say "thank you for your service," please say it with a little more meaning, a little more understanding, and a little more appreciation.

Religion

Our country was founded as a Christian nation. In 1892, in the *Church of the Holy Trinity v. the USA*, there was a unanimous decision declaring exactly that. Early patriots, Supreme Court justices, congress, and educational institutions have solidified this position. Psalm 33:12 states, "Blessed is the nation where God is the Lord."

However, our country allows for freedom of religion. We have followers of Judaism, Islam, Christianity, and various others. We also have atheists who do not believe in a supreme being. These groups are free to worship as they please. However, their objection to our well-established customs should not be allowed. The dissolution of school prayer in 1962 was an expression by our Supreme Court that the will of the majority of our people is to be ignored. This took its toll on the fabric of our society—unbelievable and unpatriotic. How about "In God We Trust"? How about a nation "Under God"? Should they go also?

Unfortunately, the leaders of some denominations have been detrimental; for example, ministers of the gospel have engaged in extramarital sex, a glaring example being the molestation of young boys by Catholic priests.

The president should take the lead to encourage religious activities, including a life of service or at least decency toward our fellow human beings.

There are things in God's world that we cannot understand; for example, exactly how did our universe originate? What is God's plan for the millions of people before Jesus—those that knew nothing about him.

Do we exist?

Infinity?

Do animals have souls? What is a soul?

Nature of heaven? Hell?

Why do bad things happen to good people?

Sacrifices?

Other space creatures?

Our responsibility to others?

I have friends that do not believe in God. I feel sorry for them. When I look at the complexities of the human body (still vastly undiscovered), the complex coloration of flowers and animals, the beauty of our forests and streams, I know that God is here.

Yes, God exists. Let us not forget it.

Even if you do not believe in a Supreme Being, consider the Ten Commandments:

1. I am the Lord thy God, thou shalt not have any strange gods before me.
2. Thou shalt not make unto thee any graven image.
3. Thou shalt not take the name of the Lord thy God in vain.
4. Remember to keep holy the Sabbath day.
5. Honor thy father and mother.
6. Thou shalt not kill.
7. Thou shalt not commit adultery.
8. Thou shalt not steal.

9. Thou shalt not bear false witness against thy
   neighbor.
10. Thou shalt not covet thy neighbor's wife; thou
    shalt not covet they neighbor's goods.

Think of the Golden Rule: "Do unto others as you would have them do unto you."

The Boy Scouts' motto: "Do a good turn daily."

Leviticus 19:18 says, "You shall love your neighbor as yourself."

Wouldn't our world be much better off if we followed these rules?

Animals

God has given us animals to enjoy, to use, and for companionship. We have eaten them, ridden them, trained them, loved them, and made them family members.

Animals have many admirable characteristics, some of which we could profit from. Animals tend to show aggression only when fearful of an attack, when their young are threatened, if hungry, or if taken by surprise. They are relentlessly devoted to their young and will defend them to death.

Many relate to humans and have become loving partners. Some have even become able to communicate with us. Dogs particularly have become wonderful partners. They are loyal to their owners, even if mistreated. They will defend their human partners to the death. Some have returned to their homes even across hundreds of miles, and others have been seen to lie next to their owners' caskets or graves until the end of their lives.

Some animals are used for food. This would not seem to contradict God's law as long as an absolute minimum of discomfort and pain is inflicted. Unfortunately, animals have also been horribly abused. They have been tortured, caged, starved, abandoned, forced to fight, or sacrificed.

Some actions are horrible and unbelievable—for example, pouring a scalding or poisonous substance onto an animal's body or shoving an object up a rectum, or setting an animal on fire. The perpetrators should not go unpunished.

If an animal is chained outside without food or water, the responsible human should be made to suffer likewise.

If an animal is shot with a bullet or arrow, the human should suffer the same action.

If an animal is beaten, exactly the same for the perpetrator.

Big game hunters—those who kill animals to stuff and hang on their walls—are among the lowest vermin of humanity. Obviously, they have no ego or self-esteem. They deserve to have their heads hanging on a wall.

Recently, a former high-level NRA executive and his wife each shot and killed a rare African elephant. This couple is despicable and pieces of s———t.

Fortunately, there are many people and organizations that help these wonderful creatures. There are feeders and protectors, companions, fundraisers, photojournalists, sanctuaries, and visitors. Cats and dogs especially have become family members that are loved and treated royally.

There was once a wonderful dog named Ralph. Ralph and his master lived on a farm outside of a city. The two were inseparable. They took hikes and swims, and Ralph particularly liked to run and chase a tennis ball.

His friend and master worked in the city and commuted. Every work day, he would return to greet Ralph, who ran down the lane and waited patiently for his return. Then he would jump up and down, and the two would return home.

One day his master was killed in a pedestrian accident in the city. Ralph ran down the lane, waiting for another joyous reunion. He waited and waited for several hours before wandering back up the lane, totally unaware of what had happened.

Every day for the rest of his life, Ralph would trot down the lane and wait for his friend. But his master would never return.

The Good

Service organizations

- Youth clubs
- Habitat for Humanity
- American Red Cross, Doctors Without Borders
- Salvation Army Boy & Girls Clubs
- Many local groups

Volunteers

- Medical
- Sports
- Disasters
- Food
- Teaching
- Environment

Companies

- Smucker's
- Bush's
- Newmar

I believe that most people are basically good. The following listing includes some of my favorites. There are many more, and I'm sure that you have many more as well.

Notable people:

- Bob Hope
- Jimmy Stewart
- Danny Thomas
- John Glenn
- John McCain
- Colin Powell
- Sister Theresa
- Oprah Winfrey
- John F. Kennedy
- Maya Angelou
- Billy Graham
- John Lewis
- Dolly Parton

Unfortunately, good people can become complacent and allow themselves to be hoodwinked by a cult leader. A prime example of this is the people of Germany in the 1940s, allowing Adolf Hitler to murder over sixteen million Jews.

Beware!

Cult

Oxford Languages definition:

> A system of religious veneration and devotion directed toward a particular figure or object.
>
> A relatively small group of people having religious beliefs or practices regarded by others as strange or sinister.
>
> A misplaced or excessive admiration for a particular person or thing. Great devotion to a person or idea.

Charles Manson, David Koresh, Jim Jones, and Adolf Hitler are examples of cult leaders. All cults have tragic endings. I suspect there is a yet undiscovered brain center in cult leaders that explains their errant actions.

Similarly, I think that the people who follow these leaders must have a cult receptive brain area that allows them to believe things that aren't true—for example, the "big lie" surrounding the 2020 election.

These people suffer from the disease "Cultitis," and there is no easy cure.

Some Random Thoughts

Let's take a poll: who has the biggest ego? Steve Harvey, Ellen DeGeneres, or Donald Trump?

Some things that really set me off:

- When you offer a friendly greeting to someone and they totally ignore you.
- When parents allow their kids to handle and break items in a store, even eat food without paying for it.

A football player and certain teammates chose to take a knee during the playing of our national anthem. Although they have the absolute right to protest for a valid cause, *patriotism must come first*. Perhaps they should be given a box lunch and parachuted into a country more to their liking.

A bad event occurs—like a mass shooting. "This must never happen again!" *It happens again.*
Another bad event occurs, perhaps similar. "This must never happen again!" *It happens again.*
Another bad event occurs, perhaps similar. "This must never happen again!" *It happens again.*
Ad nauseam…I'm sick of hearing it. Where are our responsible leaders?

Predictions

Human nature will not significantly change. There will always be the pleasant and the nasty, the good and the bad, the givers and the takers, the weak and the strong, the leaders and the followers, the rich and the poor, and then the cultists whose brains allow them to avidly follow a misguided, selfishly power-hungry egotist, even in the face of obvious truth.

Assuming there is not a nuclear holocaust that wipes out much of the civilized world, the following are predicted:

The medical field will continue to see remarkable advances. The brain will be better understood and will be able to control many body functions, and may be able to manage and cure some diseases. There will be regeneration and restoration of body parts, especially of the central nervous system, possibly eliminating paraplegia and quadriplegia. Implants will become common place and will serve various functions; they may store a person's vital information and may evolve into communication, such as phone calls.

The earth will continue to warm, and there will be more storms. Animal species will become extinct, and new disease processes will be seen. Major adjustments will have to occur since little is being done in our time.

Food habits will change. There will be less bulky but more nutritious items for consumption, and they will contain all essential nutrients. Appetite suppressants will be available. More of our water supply will come from the oceans.

Electronics will continue to affect our lives—some good, some not so good. There will be fewer human interactions, and the magical machines will continue to run our lives. There will be thinking robots.

Transportation will change dramatically. There will be personal vehicles that can travel on the land, in the air, and in the water. Subterranean tunnels will allow coast-to-coast travel in several hours. There will also be conveyances that allow for intercontinental passage deep in the seas. Space travel, already begun, will allow planetary investigation and colonization. Life will be found on other planets.

Unidentified space objects will be identified as interplanetary travel becomes commonplace. Discovery and investigation of ancient artifacts will greatly increase our knowledge of long ago.

Finally, paranormal phenomenon will allow some communication between the living and the deceased.

Some Random Thoughts

Look at the following statistics in our country, the United States of America:

1. More than 6,000 children were killed or injured by gunfire in 2022. In fact, firearms are the leading cause of death for youths ages 1 to 19.
2. The crime rate showed a 28.64 percent increase from 2019 to 2020, whereas the rate from 2018 to 2019 was only 1.19 percent.
3. In 2021, there were 16.5 violent crimes for every American aged 12 and over, and the violent crime rate was 395.7 cases per 100,000. Also, there were more than 48,000 deaths related to guns—a 23 percent increase from 9,000 in 2019.

Daily shootings, and the fear of such, have become almost routine. But we have abused our Second Amendment rights. A majority of our people are in favor of complete background checks, waiting periods, the disappearance of assault weapons, and training for permit holders.

But what have our leaders done? *Nothing.*

Democracy is defined as "a system of government by the whole population or all the eligible members of a state, typically through elected representatives."

How well are we doing?

Our elected representatives are split into two opposing factions. There is little appreciation for citizen welfare (e.g., a majority of our people desire strong yet reasonable gun control). But no action.

Unethical practices, dishonesty, and sexual indiscretion are common, affecting many leaders, even in the Supreme Court.

Trillions of dollars are spent on political ballyhoo yet many important projects are underfunded, and many citizens are left without food or housing.

We spend trillions of dollars on space exploration before addressing our earthly problems (e.g., decaying structures, health concerns, the environment, and education).

We have no policy on border control.

We have multiple millionaires and even billionaires, most of whom do not pay their fair share due to tax loopholes and legal shenanigans

Although our country professes to be "a nation under God," there seems to be less and less emphasis on religion.

Is our democracy being threatened by cultism, egotism, immorality, and lies?

As previously discussed, sex (sexual intercourse) should occur between two individuals for the purpose of procreation and for committed loving intimacy.

Perhaps you think that sex in other situations should not occur. Indeed, if that were so,

- many unwanted children would not be born, lessening childhood psychological damage, and the burden on the biological parents;
- the overpopulation problem would be lessened;
- fewer demands would be made on tax dollars;
- the rates of venereal diseases—such as gonorrhea, syphilis, and HIV—would plummet; and
- abortion would be less of a consideration.

Are you really advocating sex in this manner, you say?

Yes!

We love music! There is rock, R & B, country, jazz, heavy metal, Soul, folk, disco, and verbal diarrhea known as hiphop. We tend to admire certain performers while jumping up and down, shouting, and waving our arms in excitement as we watch them perform contortions, hear the loud noise that causes hearing problems in later life, and of course the various hairdos, the torn clothing, and the lifting of a leg as if to pee on a fireplug.

Certain performers become "stars" who attain notoriety and wealth. We tend to think of them as talented people, even though many people could perform just as well if they had the desire and training and possibly a lucky break.

However, if you would like to experience real talent, listen to symphonies by Bach, Mendelson, Tchaikovsky,

Mozart, Beethoven, Chopin, and others. Piano concertos reveal a career of total dedication. These people have a lifetime of long daily practice and experience in classical groups. They strive for perfection and exhibit true talent.

Regarding the drug problem in our country...

If we didn't use them, there would be no problem with trafficking and cartels!

Most deaths from high doses of illicit drugs are not "accidental overdoses"; they are suicides.

Obesity is the most pressing health problem in our country today.

Before we have a problem with *Black* people, we should recall several centuries ago it was *White* people who tore families apart and made slaves of family members.

Thin ties, wide ties, long pants, short pants, crewcut, dreadlocks, tattoos, nose rings, and now beards growing on males, most of which tend to be scraggly with multiple colors and lengths, unkempt, and just plain ugly. What's next?

Beware of advertisements, especially on television. Many are misleading, inaccurate, and even dishonest. Don't be fooled!

We have made considerable progress in the fight against animal cruelty by making dog racing illegal. How about horses?

Electronics

Electronics have taken over. We are able to talk to almost anyone at any time, we can obtain information nearly instantaneously, we can call for assistance, we can monitor, we can calculate, and we can take photos.

On the other hand, we can send pictures of our genitals and embarrassing activities for all to see. We can annoy other people, walk into glass doors while looking at phones, and cause traffic accidents resulting in injuries and deaths.

Scamming is becoming commonplace.

The trend has just begun. Artificial intelligence is going to change many things in the future. It's possible that we could be subjects of robots.

Author Facts

1. Grew up in a small town
2. Eagle Scout
3. College and doctoral degree
4. Retired AF officer
5. Served in health-care field for over fifty years